Basketball Diet

Winning Eating Habits for Basketball Games and Life

by

David Smith

B180 Basketball, Inc.
P.O. Box 2406
Midland, MI 48641-2406
www.b180basketball.com
Phone: 1-800-957-1275

Published by B180 Basketball, Inc. 6-3-18

ISBN: 978-1-7325361-3-5 (sc)
ISBN: 978-1-7325361-2-8 (e)

Library of Congress Control Number: 2018943470

Contents

Dedication

This book is dedicated to my mother, the late Connie Smith and my father, the late David C. Smith Sr., and all of my siblings. I love you always.

Acknowledgments

I'd like to acknowledge all the coaches, trainers, and health professionals that have played a part in my development and awareness of living a health-conscious lifestyle. I wasn't perfect, but I gave my best and learned from my mistakes. Thank you.

Introduction

Dieting has been an important part of the success or failure of basketball players throughout their careers. Whether it's a middle school athlete or a seasoned professional basketball player, the role that a diet plays is key to their future success. How an individual prepares their body for the next stage or chapter in their life involves choosing the right food to eat. There are many instances in towns across the United States that you will see the following scenario play out. There's a basketball tournament going on. Players, young and old, wake up early. They'll eat cereal that's full of sugar, a ham or sausage breakfast sandwich, or a breakfast bar that may be high in sugar. They may choose to eat another high sugar breakfast snack and fruit such as a banana, orange, or apple. Finally, they will drink a sports drink, soda, a glass of milk, or orange juice. Then off to the tournament. What's wrong with this, you may be asking? Well, the amount of sugar and other bad ingredients that are in the food that's consumed has made what looks like a good start to a day, in all actuality, really bad. That is; bad for the long-term health of the person. The amount of sugar in this instance is very high. So are the amount of calories that are consumed. You might be thinking right now, they are about to participate in a basketball tourney and will sweat off the calories. That's true. However, once they get to the tourney, there are other food options that are presented to the individual throughout the day, such as pizza, hot dogs, hamburger, pretzels, fries, various peanuts, popcorn, and more high sugar beverages. How can a person truly make a rational decision on what food to consume if the food that is truly bad for you is at the forefront the majority of the time? The reason this book was written is to provide a plan of action for basketball players and athletes when choosing what to eat, regardless of which stage of career they are at.

The focus of the book is to use the plan of action that is created to help maximize on-court performance while also reaching long-term personal health and longevity goals as it relates to healthy eating and living.

How to use this book:

Read the section that corresponds to your situation. Create a plan of action with the help of the information in this book, your trainers, and support team (coach, dietitian, etc.) Stay positive and motivated to reach your personal and long-term health goals.

Note: The views in this book are the author's views. For additional information on dieting or exercise, you can get resources and information from your health care provider.

Five Habits to Defeat as a Basketball Player

- Late Night Eating
- Sugar, Sugar, Sugar
- Chips, Fries, and Pizza
- Large Portions and Second Helpings
- Alcohol and Drugs

Late Night Eating

Fast but unhealthy. The temptation to eat late at night is enhanced the later a person stays awake. From TV commercials to online ads about food, cravings for something to eat takes over an individual's thoughts. In most cases, what's normally available to eat at home isn't enough. The individual seeks complete gratification. So, he or she embarks on an adventure to find a restaurant or fast food place to satisfy their hunger. If the individual is already out on the town late at night, then the potential for sporadic eating is increased and eating unhealthy food late at night can destroy any workout or long-term personal goals. Over time, the instant gratification a person receives from satisfying their cravings for food is met with unwanted weight gain, fatigue & laziness, overeating, and damaged self-esteem.

Wasting Money

The amount of money that is spent late at night on food, snacks, and beverages add up. If a person were to add the total cost of what they spent on late night food, it would come as a shock to them. Let's take for example an individual goes to a late night fast food restaurant. The individual spends on average seven dollars on a value meal. They then go to a local convenience store and spends an additional three dollars on snacks. If the individual eats late night food four times a week, this would total up to $40 spent on late night eating. What if the individual did this for a year? Considering there's 52 weeks in a year, that would be about $2,080 annually. If the individual continues to eat out consistently at the same pace, the person in 10 years would have spent $20,800 on late night foods and snacks. This money could be used or invested to serve a better purpose. When deciding to spend on late night food, consider the long-term financial effects.

Role Models

Picture this. A young fan has followed his favorite basketball player's journey since high school. The fan mimics everything the basketball player does. The fan even eats, talks, and dresses like their favorite basketball player. The young fan has ambitions and plans to teach their children and others that they will have influence over in the future the exact same strategies they learned from their favorite basketball player. Is this situation good? What long-term effects does the gradual or sudden weight gain of an athlete have on their fans and followers?

As a role model, basketball players at every level of competition must consider the effects of their eating habits because there is some little fan out there watching their every move, on and off the basketball court. When an athlete embraces the true uniqueness of the power that they hold to influence the youths of the next generation in a good way, they will continuously strive to improve themselves off the court in all aspects of life. Monitoring when and what a basketball player eats for breakfast, lunch, and dinner is important for game competition. A basketball player who's in a role model position must know that someone wants to be just like them. This should have an effect on the choices of what's consumed and what not.

Goals

When a basketball player is training, regardless of whether its off-season or in-season, there are developed goals that he strives to attain. These goals were put in place to get better physically, mentally, and skillfully.

The effect that late-night eating has on an individual's goal attainment is something to monitor. If an individual chooses to follow their workout routine during the day only to eat and add food that's high in sugar, sodium, calories, and fat at night, it keeps the individual from seeing any consistent gain towards reaching their goal. They constantly have to start over. Instead, the basketball player should practice developing a clear goal to eliminate late night eating. This will, in turn, help the individual reach their maximum potential during training sessions.

Form a New Habit

In order to form new habits that help to stop late night eating, self-awareness must be acknowledged by the basketball player. They must understand that pizza is not Ok at 3:30 am in the morning, two or three times every week. Alternative options that can be put in place to stop late night eating are:

1. Keep a Budget and Limit Spending
2. Eat Fruit or Low Sugar and Calorie Foods
3. Only Water
4. Small Portion Sizes
5. Find an Accountability Partner

A description of each alternative option follows.

Keep a Budget and Limit Spending

The amount of money spent on late night eating on a daily, weekly, monthly, and annual basis is monitored. This option requires a person to set a spending limit and follow it strategically. For example, an individual sets their monthly spending limit on late night spending to forty dollars or ten dollars a week. To make sure that the spending limit is kept and honored, leave all credit cards and bank cards at home when you go out to eat late at night. Use cash to pay for everything. Spending limits should be set at two to five percent of your monthly income, or lower. It should not be higher than the amount that you donate to worthy causes on a monthly or annual basis.

Eat Fruit or Low Sugar and Calorie Foods

Choosing fruit, low sugar, or low-calorie food options are better than eating fast food or food from restaurants late at night. Two bananas and an apple along with a stick of string cheese should satisfy a person's hunger. Eating a fruit, low calorie, and low sugar options keep the individual on track to reach their training or workout goals. The cost of the fruit and string cheese also fits into any spending limit that would be created. There are many combinations of fruit, cheese, and other low sugar food options to pick from. If you know that you are going to eat late at night for several days in a given week, create a menu of the fruit, low sugar, and low-calorie food options that you want to eat.

Only Water

When up late at night, the simple solution to prevent adding unwanted calories to a late-night meal is to drink only water. Pop or soda is high in calories and sugar. Energy drinks are high in caffeine, sugar, and other ingredients that your body can do without that late at night. Drinking water keeps your body hydrated and on pace to reach training goals.

Small Portion Sizes

If you happen to eat out late at a restaurant or fast food place, eat a small portion of the meal and either give the rest away or throw it away. Don't take it with you because you will be tempted to eat the remainder of the food. Choosing to eat small portions limit the amount of calories you take in. The fast food still may be unhealthy for you. The underlying goal here is to not overeat and pack on unwanted calories.

Find an Accountability Partner

An accountability partner can be a friend, relative, trainer, or someone you trust. Having a partner who understands your goals and long-term plans will benefit you when you're out late at night at social events. They will help keep most situations such as overeating, drinking pop, soda, or alcohol under control. Communicate clearly to your accountability partner your plans before you arrive at the event. This will clear up any misunderstandings.

As a young boy, I witnessed the negative effects that late-night eating has on a person, first hand. My father was a great man. He worked seven days a week and most of the time, twelve hours a day. He'd normally go to work at 2 pm and would either get home at 12 am or 2 am. When he got home, he would eat a huge meal that was prepared by my mother. I'm talking chicken, steak, or pork chops, macaroni & cheese, cornbread, dressing, corn, baked beans and collard greens type of meal. He would then drink his coffee, smoke a cigarette or two then go to bed. Over a ten-year period, this type of eating and way of life takes a toll on anyone. His body began to break down rapidly. Ultimately, the late-night eating and cigarettes got the best of him. To me, my father will always be Superman. Use his story to create a change in your late-night eating habits. It will make all the difference in the world to someone who cares about you.

Sugar, Sugar, Sugar

Look around at the food products in a store. Look at what someone is eating right now. The ingredient, sugar, is in almost every food item offered. It's in fast food items. It's even in soup. The everyday food that's consumed by individuals such as cereal, breakfast bars, sports drinks, and baked desserts are very high in sugar content. Individuals rarely take the time to ask someone for information or look for themselves at the number of grams of sugar that's in what they are about to eat. By failing to do this, the overall consumption of sugar on a daily basis is increased to a high level.

The high amount of sugar that's consumed on a daily basis, if not monitored, can cause a person to feel tired, have headaches, have unwanted weight gain, and develop long-term heart problems. It also causes a person to eventually lose their teeth. Why risk overloading your body with high amounts of sugar if there are harmful effects? You might be thinking or saying to yourself, "Because it tastes so good. That's why!" Well, yes, you are right. You can still experience a gratifying experience by just educating yourself on finding and using healthier options to replace the sugar ingredient in the food that you consume.

Curbing a craving for candy may seem like a hard task for someone. To start out, try looking at the candy wrapper and actually find out how many grams of sugar are in the candy that you are about to eat. If this doesn't shock you or change your mind, begin to educate yourself on and compare the amount of sugar content found in candy or the food you like to eat. Then search for similar candy options with less sugar in it. Over time, your craving for the high sugar candy will diminish because of your awareness of its content and the education you've gained of alternative options.

Resisting cakes, pies, and muffins is a challenge. For example, you might have your favorite cake that's made for you by a loved one. Then there's your favorite dessert to eat after work or on the way home. Get an understanding of what ingredients are included in the making of the desserts that you like to eat. Develop a plan to eliminate the everyday consumption of these types of desserts. Alternative ingredient options could be used to eliminate the amount of sugar you consume. You might be asking at this point, what alternative sugar options are there? Honey, fruit, or any other naturally sweet option should be considered. Naturally sweet alternatives are better for your body. When choosing a sports drink or soda pop, consider the amount of sugar that is in the drink. There may be instant thirst-quenching gratification initially. However, when it matters most, the sugar that you've consumed will eventually conquer you if you do not conquer and control sugar first.

As a basketball coach, I found myself eating unintentionally unhealthy most of the time. I clearly remember how a typical day as a coach would go. I'd wake up early and go to lift weights and exercise at the gym. After exercising, I'd get a coffee, energy drink, a breakfast sandwich, and a donut. I'd then head to work. During the day at lunchtime, I'd eat a big lunch because I knew that I was going to miss dinner. So, lunch would typically consist of a footlong sub, a bag of chips, a muffin, and a lemonade. By the time practice was about to start, I'd eat cookies, a candy bar, or something sweet. I'd then stand and watch as practice took place. On the way home, I'd get another sports drink or soda pop and another donut, breakfast bar, or candy bar (What I ate on a typical day as a former college basketball player would be similar to when I was coaching. I would have increased the amount of sugar foods eaten daily). After analyzing my eating habits and lack of physical activity during the day while at work and at practice, I realized that by eliminating foods that contained sugar from my diet and including walking and running in my exercise plan would prepare me for good health in the long term. Initially, I took sugar completely out of my diet and replaced sugar cravings with honey and different fruits. If I had an extreme sweet craving, I ate fruit. Normally two bananas and an apple or pear.

Chips, Fries, and Pizza

At a young age, a person is hooked on the mouth-watering taste of chips, French fries, and pizza. Lunchtime at most middle and high schools across the United States has cafeterias offering these food options. Various types of potato chips fill the vending machines in the school hallways. Used as a daily snack food, these items have become the meal of choice for students most days. Take a deep look, and you will find that these food choices are very bad for an individual. The high sodium, lack of nutrients, and high-fat content all play a damaging role in destroying the health and body of an individual. If a young person is trying to prepare for a basketball season as well as for life after the season, then choosing food that will increase their overall performance and health level should be the option.

The obesity rate in today's youths and adults are to some extent caused by the overeating of chips, fries, and pizza. What should an individual do? It's quick, sometimes cheap, and it tastes good. Yes, this is too good to be true. The long-term effects of continuing to eat this type of food, day after day can lead to major health problems such as heart failure and diabetes. Individuals are not able to reach personal or sports specific performance goals consistently if they continue to eat these foods.

Alternative options include food that's low in sugar, sodium, and calories. The food should not be greasy or fried. It must provide nutrients that the body needs on a daily basis. An example would be eating dried fruit and a low-fat sub sandwich. It's a sacrifice, but if nothing is put in place, disaster will be the end result.

You see it year after year. On road trips, basketball tournaments, and at team parties; they are filled with chips, fries, and pizza. To change the course of a person's future, action must be taken. Making a food sacrifice will come with some drawbacks because you are not able to eat just anything. However, there are more positive results, long-term. A person's body must be cared for. It's the only body you'll get in a lifetime. The overall focus is not to eliminate eating this food completely but eating in moderation. What does moderation mean, you may ask? For this book's definition, it means eating a particular food one to three times a month only. If a person is able to completely eliminate chips, fries, and pizza from their diet, reaching personal long-term goals and game performance goals will begin to align in a positive way.

As a high school basketball player, I remember some days eating only a large French fry for the entire day. This was by choice. I didn't take the time to truly analyze the long-term effects of eating that way. Across the United States, there are individuals currently choosing to eat this way by choice. Awareness of alternative food choices and a commitment to learning to read and understand food labels will improve the eating habits of individuals, young and old.

Large Portions and Second Helpings

It may have started with a dish made by your grandmother. You ate bite after bite and was experiencing pure satisfaction. The thought never occurred that too much food would cause harm to the body. As you know, people tend to eat more of something that tastes good. People even purposefully over eat when participating in an eating contest. Whether seen on TV, Social Media, or in Person, eating large portions of food or second helpings can cause weight gain and other health complications. The long-term effect of eating large portions may lead to heart disease. The thought process of an individual that chooses to eat a second helping of mashed potatoes and gravy may not be totally aware of what the additional food will actually do to their body. The individual is just satisfying an immediate craving. You see this at holiday time. Uncontrollable consumption of large portions of food and continuously going back for second helpings. Maybe most of us got this from our parents telling us to eat everything on our plates. Maybe we got this from there not being enough food to go around in the family. Either way, when no consciousness is given to making a decision on whether to eat more food or not, overeating, nausea, and weight gain occur. In the United States, large portion size servings of food items on a plate or meal are the norm for most restaurants and other social gatherings. The informed and knowledgeable person will use caution when dining out or eating at social gatherings. What about the uninformed person? What are they to do? To start, they must become aware of the situation and what options they have. If a person chooses to wait too long in the day before they decide to eat anything, they will be met with an overindulgence of the food that they eat. When athletes and coaches are on road trips or at tournaments filling up at an all-you-can-eat buffet, they must be aware of what they choose to eat and how much of it to eat. To change this way of eating, a person must follow the guidelines that are set forth in their diet or training plan.

Stick to the plan, no matter what. Overcome the urge to eat everything on your plate by discarding a portion of the food before you initially eat or request a smaller portion size.

I remember as a young boy, I loved when my family got pizza to eat. I'd try to eat about seven or eight pieces myself. The pizza normally had everything except anchovies on them too. I just remember after eating that last piece I felt horrible. It still tasted good, but I didn't take the time to actually realize that I was purposely hurting myself. It's been a long time since those days. I am now a knowledgeable person and lifelong learner that strives to better myself daily and to assist others in reaching their ultimate goals. I now maintain a strategy to control what and how much I eat by choosing to eat small portion sizes when dining out or eating at other social gatherings the majority of the time.

Alcohol and Drugs

"It won't hurt you" is normally the words that's spoken by a friend to someone that's about to experience alcohol or drugs for the first time. People who choose to use alcohol and drugs become depressed and sometimes aloof. They hurt the individuals that love them most by not listening to them. It's like God sending down a special angel picked out just for you and you ignore everything the angel tells you. Deliver on the dream that you promised yourself. Hanging out with the wrong type of friends is the base root of the problem. Your mind will tell you that it's ok, but it's really not. Challenge yourself to do more in life. Whatever happened in the past won't change. The only thing that matters is the current moment and your future choices. The use of alcohol and drugs limits the mind of what it truly can accomplish. You must ask yourself, how can a person lead his followers if they don't have control of their own mind and their own mind is less than half developed? You have a gift to give to the world. Without the complete use of your mind, that gift will remain dormant. If given the chance, your mind will set your life free. The lack of belief by those of limited faith and security has caused a full reliance on alcohol and drugs as a remedy. This is a trap that only those who develop their minds realize. Those who rely on alcohol and drugs to get by in life are cursed with constant deceptions of false realities. Overcoming this requires commitment to a permanent change.

Let's look at for example a basketball player that develops the habit of smoking marijuana while in high school. The basketball player then chooses to continue using the drug in college and at a more frequent pace. The effect that marijuana has on the player initially seems minor or non-existent. A closer look at the situation will show that the basketball player's mind/brain has been crippled. They begin to lose the battle of gaining control of their own mind. They slowly become less dependent on their brain and ability to truly think. This puts the basketball player behind, compared to the average person at their same age that doesn't do drugs. The only way to change this is to become aware of the effects of drugs and quit using drugs instantly. Then start developing your mind.

Look at your life. Remember where you have been and know where you are going. In your past, there may have been a friend or relative that had a strong dependence on alcohol and/or drugs. You saw firsthand how their life was destroyed. Use their experience as a lesson to change your life. Alcohol such as beer, wine, gin, vodka, cognac, etc. and all drugs (marijuana, prescription drugs, cocaine, crack, heroin, etc.) will let you win the first few rounds. A person may feel that nothing is wrong or happening to them, and it's ok. Then all of a sudden, the mind and body breaks down. In the later rounds, alcohol and drugs win. They are undefeated. To win the battle, follow your basketball and life goals. Eliminate the dependence on alcohol and drugs for life. Your family, children, future grandchildren, friends, the people who love you back, and your fans are counting on you.

As a young boy, I saw firsthand the effects that drinking alcohol and using drugs has on a person. I saw neighbors, friends, and family die inside. Though they were still living physically, their purpose for living died. Their mind and body were taken. In turn, they became permanently dependent on alcohol and/or drugs. This hurt me inside because as a friend or relative, I wasn't able to change their decisions. The final decision to drink alcohol or use drugs rests solely on the individual. They must not make impulse decisions while in the moment. Take a minute to truly think about your long-term goals and plans for your life.

Chapter 1

Chapter 1
Family History: Home Cooking

Looking back at a time in your past, you may remember when your family and friends gathered for a large feast. The food that was served seemed to be made just right. There may have been an unlimited supply of your favorite food dish. Being the official taste tester was the chosen title you may have had. That is, before the food was actually done cooking, you tasted it for quality. Family gatherings are a time when history is made. Traditions are passed down to the younger generations. Special recipes are shared. Prayers are made. Ways of living and eating are shared. The unique time that is shared with family can't be taken for granted. There is laughter as well as pain that molds a person into who they are as an individual and who they will become. The food that is eaten, especially during holidays, reflect culture, religion, and traditions from past ancestors. As a basketball player and athlete, the decisions that you make regarding what to eat and what family traditions to continue have a lasting effect on the next generation. Careful consideration must be given to keep your family traditions alive but in a healthier and life-saving way. What I mean by this is think about using healthy alternative ingredients when preparing traditional family meals.

Deciding what's good for you to eat in family gatherings is difficult. Limiting the amount of sugar-heavy foods and beverages is a good start. Enjoy your favorite foods but in small portion sizes. There's a tendency to eat more at family gatherings. It's easy to lose track of what you've actually eaten because you may be sidetracked by the presence of family members that you haven't seen in a while. Consideration must be taken for the short and long-term training and dieting goals that you have planned out. An average daily intake of calories could be 2,000 calories. This could be surpassed in one sitting at family gatherings. Overeating at family gatherings causes your calorie intake to skyrocket. I remember when I was a little boy. I loved helping my grandmother and mother prepare food. Like you may think of your grandmother and mother, I believe that they cook the best soul food in the world. I'm talking chicken, ham, turkey, dressing, greens, cornbread, homemade mac n cheese, chitlins, corn on the cob, baked beans, potato salad, black-eyed peas, ham hocks, saltwater cornbread, etc. mmmm mmmm mmmm. They made everything from scratch too. So, they needed a taste tester. I gladly volunteered! The ingredients used to prepare these foods can be high in sodium, sugar, and fat. The portion sizes can cause for a large intake of calories as well. When it came time for family gathering, as I got older, I had to limit the portion sizes of the food that I ate as well as to stop eating certain foods such as pork and shrimp altogether. I stopped eating all kinds of pork and shrimp because I felt as animals or creatures, what they ate to survive did not coincide with what I wanted in my own body. I became more mindful of my long-term health goals as it related to preparing to compete in basketball games. I also began to think of others and extreme situations. For example, what happens when there is no parent to cook daily meals? What happens when a family is homeless? There are issues and situations that will affect the life of an athlete or coach. Seeking help from food pantries, shelters, and other family and friends may be a short-term solution. Don't feel down and out because of this. Just stay positive and create a detailed plan to better your situation day by day. Have faith, pray, and stick to your plan. When you have to cook for yourself and others, learn to use healthy alternatives for ingredients. This will have a major effect on how future generations develop and carry on your family traditions. Be mindful of what you say about how food tastes. Your family members and friends are listening to you, and they may be trying to be like you. So, if you don't like a certain food item and you say it aloud, they may decide not to like it too. Teach future generations the importance of reading food labels, watching sugar and salt intake, and monitoring their daily calorie intake. Explain the short and long-term effects as it relates to sports competition and life. If you are able and blessed to do this, hire a chef that prepares daily meals using a careful process. Strive to keep family traditions alive but in a healthier version. The chef should be very conscious of healthy foods and dieting trends for sports competition. They should also understand coaches' and retired athletes' lifestyles. The chef should be able to prepare meals that carry on family traditions as well as prepare low sugar, sodium, and calorie food options. The beverages that are prepared and consumed should also be low in these categories.

Chapter 2

Chapter 2
Establishing Goals for Eating Healthy

Take a look at yourself in the mirror. Are you happy with your outside appearance? Next, go to the doctor and have a complete physical examination done. Are you happy with your current physical and health status? When you begin to establish goals for eating healthy, you must first analyze your current physical fitness level and overall health. If you are not happy and satisfied with your current results, you must decide what would make you happy as it pertains to your physical fitness level and overall health. Then map out a plan to reach the goal of making yourself happy. The plan that you design should outline the changes that you make to your daily habits. It should provide a detail explanation of where you want to be from a physical fitness standpoint and overall health at the same time next year. A detail explanation should also be done for a five and ten-year outlook. When making in-season and out of season dieting goals and plans, consider factors such as late-night practices, social events, banquets, and game days. How do you plan to monitor your results? What if you fail and eat everything that's unhealthy for you? These questions will come up often. This book will help you answer them. Treat your plans and goals that you make like a practice plan. Write out your strategies daily as you would when creating a practice or workout plan. Then follow the plan that you create. Just like in basketball practice, you won't perform the drill to perfection the first time. It takes repetition. What follows are examples of sample healthy eating goals for in season, out of season, basketball players, coaches, retired basketball players & coaches, and lifelong health.

Note: The examples that follow are the authors' views. When planning meals, seek assistance from a dietician or other professionals.

Goals for Eating Healthy- In Season:

- Eat two different types of nuts daily

- Eat low sugar, calorie, and sodium foods after games

- Use no illegal drugs and stay away from negative influences

- Follow daily and weekly meal plans created by you or your dietitian (reach 80% of planned meal consumption)

- Eat chips and other similar types of snack foods one to two times per week

- Limit dependence on over the counter and prescription drugs (use only if needed or emergency)

- Eat at least two different types of fruits daily

- Eat at least two different types of grains daily

- Drink at least two liters of water daily

- Eat at least three cups of different types of vegetables daily

Goals for Eating Healthy- Out of Season:

- Follow daily and weekly meal plans created by yourself or your dietitian

- Adjust your plan according to your goal of wanting to either gain or lose weight

- Do not use any type of illegal drug and stay away from negative influences

- Limit your dependence on over the counter and prescription drugs to an only if needed or emergency situation

Goals for Eating Healthy- For Basketball Players:

- Eat meat or fish that's low in fat

- Do not eat late at night (after 10 pm)

- Limit the eating of snack foods and food that is high in sugar and sodium
- Drink Milk
- Drink Water
- Take a multivitamin daily
- Eat light at banquets and buffets
- Eat at least three servings of pasta weekly
- Eat three different vegetables daily
- Eat three different fruits daily
- Eat light before practices and games (at least one and a half hour before)

Goals for Eating Healthy- For Coaches:

- Do not eat late at night (after 10 pm)
- Limit the eating of snack foods and food that is high in sugar and sodium
- Do not drink beverages that are high in caffeine (no more than one daily)
- Eat a low-fat dinner before practice and games
- Eat three different vegetables daily
- Eat three different fruits daily
- Take a multivitamin daily
- Eat two different types of nuts daily
- Eat light at banquets and buffets
- Drink green tea

Goals for Eating Healthy- Retired Basketball Players and Coaches:

- Do not eat late at night (after 10 pm)
- Limit snack foods and foods that are high in sugar and sodium
- Do not eat candy (if needed, eat no sugar added candy)
- Eat low sugar dessert options
- Eat three different vegetables daily
- Eat three different fruits daily
- Take a multivitamin daily
- Do not drink energy drinks
- Eat a breakfast that's low in fat, sugar, and sodium
- Eat two different types of nuts daily

Goals for Eating Healthy- Lifelong Health

- Do not eat late at night (after 10 pm)
- Limit snack foods and food high in fat, sugar, sodium, and calories
- Eat three different vegetables daily
- Eat three different fruits daily
- Take a multivitamin daily
- Eat two different types of nuts daily
- Drink Milk
- Drink Water
- Eat breakfast daily
- Eat meat or fish that is lean and low in fat
- Follow and adjust your meal plan based on your goals to either maintain or lose weight

Stay committed to your overall health goals. There will be outside influences that will attempt to deter you from your plan. A simple smell of certain foods may trigger an eat everything moment. If this happens, and it will, bounce back with a renewed effort to better your last attempt. Remember, your ultimate end goal is to make yourself happy with your physical fitness level and overall health.

Chapter 3

Chapter 3
Eating Food During the Season

For Basketball Players:

As the season goes on, there will be several opportunities to develop and practice good eating habits. Avoiding snack food and unhealthy beverages will be a continuous challenge. Keep your short and long-term goals in mind. Take the time to truly analyze where you are currently and where it is that you want to go.

For Coaches:

Long days full of practices, film sessions, scouting, recruiting, scheduling, and planning takes a toll on a coach's body. Snack foods, energy drinks, and most fast food should be avoided over the course of the season. There will be times that eating unhealthy food is the only option. It is at that moment when a conscious decision must be made to seek and find an alternative food option.

Whether you are a coach or basketball player, what you eat before and after practice should be planned out. Most of the time, it's an in the moment decision that is made to grab junk food. There normally is no involvement to think or read the package labels on the food that's bought. Eat at least an hour and a half before practice. Fruit and vegetables should be included in whatever you choose to eat. After practice meals should follow the diet plan that you create. If your practices are late (say 8 pm-10 pm), then you should have already eaten dinner before 6:30 pm. The urge will be present to eat after practice. Choose low sugar, low calorie, and low-fat food options. The strategy outlined above should also be used when eating food before and after basketball games.

Team and family functions during the season will often have food options present that are full of fat, sugar, and sodium. It's like you are attending a holiday gathering. Be mindful of what food you consume and how much of it. Don't overeat. Choose to eat the healthiest food options that are available. The team and family functions that I'm referring to are team parties, birthday parties, team building events (example: bowling), and family reunions. There may be other events and functions that can be considered a team or family function as well. Eating at travel basketball tournaments would fall into the category of a team function.

Scouting and recruiting trips done by coaches are long and demanding days. The food that is chosen to eat on road trips should be similar to what is chosen when traveling with the entire team. Choose food options such as low-fat sub sandwiches, fruit, veggies, and a low sugar beverage to eat. This will help you maintain a health-conscious lifestyle. Your awareness and overall mood can be affected by what you eat. As a coach or player, it's important to keep a positive state of mind. Listed below are some examples of food options to provide strength and energy, increase stamina, support the mind, and help the body recover from athletic competition.

Note: The food options listed are the authors' views. Talk to your dietitian or other professional for additional information.

Food Options for Strength and Energy:

Bananas	Walnuts/Other Nuts and Seeds
Beans	Apricots
Raisins	Chias
Lean Meats	Avocados
Eggs	Brown Rice
Water	Milk
Kale	Acai Berries
Spinach/Leafy Greens	Watermelon
Tuna/Salmon/Other Fish	Broccoli
Cottage Cheese	Yogurt

Apples	

Food Options To Increase or Maintain Stamina:

Fish	Cherries
Eggs	Sweet Potatoes
Milk	Kale
Barley	Bananas
Oatmeal	Red Peppers
Watermelon Blueberries	Carrots
Walnuts/Other Nuts & Seeds	Lean Meats
Apples	Beets
Soy	Coconut Water
Almonds	

Food Options to Support the Mind:

Blueberries	Brown Rice
Salmon/Other Fish	Beans
Nuts and Seeds	Dark Chocolate
Avocados	Unsweetened Brewed Tea
Oatmeal	Spinach/Leafy Greens
Milk	Celery
Oranges/Other Citrus Fruits	Rice
Whole Grains	Barley
Lean Meats	Soy
Yogurt	Pomegranates
Broccoli	

Food Options To help The Body Recover from Competition:

Yogurt	Beets
Cottage Cheese	Ginger
Milk/Dairy Foods	Oranges/Grapefruits/Citrus Fruits
Eggs	Carrots
Fish or Other Lean Meat	Squash
Nuts and Seeds	Blueberries/Cherries/Dark Fruits
Beans	Cauliflower and Broccoli
Spinach/Leafy Greens	Sweet Potatoes
Mushrooms	Watermelon
Green Tea	Almonds
Soy	Bok Choy

The sample food options listed above is just that, a sample. There are more options available. I encourage you to find out what foods will help you to reach your individual health, fitness, basketball, and lifelong goals. Read the food labels on the items you purchase. Understand that there will be times when you do not make the right choices as it pertains to eating food. Bounce back from failures and start again. You will be successful.

Chapter 4

Chapter 4
Eating Food During the Off-Season

At this point, you should have established off-season goals that will be your guide. View the goals that you establish daily. This will help keep the goals fresh in your mind. When considering a goal, determine the long-term effect it will have on your life as well as your upcoming season. The goals should not be limited to dieting. It should include fitness & weight training and basketball skill workout goals. The food that is eaten before training workouts should be light and done at least an hour and a half before the training session. Breakfast is the most important meal, so don't skip this meal! Light fruit, yogurt, or some other low fat, low sugar, and low-calorie food option should be eaten. Remember to take a daily multivitamin as well.

Holiday gatherings and parties during the off-season will be a test of your commitment level to the goals that you have established. Be cautious of the food choices at these gatherings. Don't be afraid to ask the host about the ingredients used to make a certain food item that you want to eat. The temptation to eat unhealthy items will be increased by the people that are around you. They will say, "One piece won't hurt you." In reality, it will damage your commitment and overall focus to your plan.

Alcohol and drugs will be a constant exposure throughout your journey. The quick joy and satisfaction that you receive after consumption are paid for later on down the line. If you can imagine yourself in a boxing match. Your opponent is alcohol and drugs. You are scheduled to go 12 rounds (Your lifespan). You may win the first few rounds. However, the body blows that are delivered by alcohol and drugs over the course of every round ultimately defeats you by the time the 12th round (old age/end of career) occurs. Choose wisely when making decisions about drug use. Stay away from negative people, negative social events, and other negative influences.

Monitor your progress during the off-season. Knowing what you ate over the course of the week, and how many workouts you attended will help keep you on track to reach your off-season goals.

Chapter 5

Chapter 5
Eating Food at Social Events

Overeating is a common occurrence at social events. It starts with the appetizer and ends with the unlimited number of beverages consumed. If both of your hands are tied when deciding on what to eat, choose the healthiest option available. Peer pressure will be there. Friends and family will suggest that you should try certain foods or say that you've always eaten certain foods. Social events are a trap. You have the best of both worlds. Everyone that you want to see and everything that you want to eat are there. The more you are able to resist temptation and stick to your goals and plans, the more self-disciplined as a person you will become. The challenge that you will most commonly face is defending your stance on what you choose to eat or not eat.

After you have been drinking alcohol or smoking marijuana, there is an enhanced temptation to eat. Most of the time, the first food item you will notice is a dessert. Say no to this temptation and instead, choose a healthier food option as well as drink as much water as you can. Discuss your diet with those that are close to you or another supportive friend. That way, you have someone who will help you in your time of need. I've always found it difficult to eat food at a funeral. I understand that at some funerals, the religion of the deceased person and the members of the church may coincide the death as a celebration. A sort of going home. They will prepare a meal for the family members. Whether you choose to eat or not at any type of social event, don't let your emotions make you overeat. It's better to avoid all unhealthy food at social events because one bite won't be enough. Eating only vegetables, fruit, lean meats, cheese, and drinking water will be a safer option to keep you on track to reach your short and long-term health goals.

Chapter 6

Chapter 6
Shopping for Food

Low Fat, Low Sugar, Low Calorie, Low Sodium

When Shopping for food and groceries, have a clear plan in mind. Look at your goals that you have created. The goals can be basketball specific, health related, or fitness related. As you analyze your short and long-term goals, write a list down of foods that you can eat that will help you reach them. The list that you make will be separate from your shopping list. When you decide to create a shopping list, take into consideration the cost of the foods that you intend to purchase and your budget. The budget that you have may vary week to week or month to month. The objective is to buy the right food at the right price. Reading the labels on the food that you purchase is very important. It will help you become smart as well as an informed buyer. Knowing how many calories, sugar, sodium, and fat grams that are in the food that you purchase is important. Choose food items that are low in these categories. That is, shop for low calorie, low sugar, low sodium, and low-fat food items. This may sound like it's tough and time-consuming. Once you check the labels on the food that you are about to purchase a few times, you will remember them and get used to it.

Produce Aisle First

When you begin to shop for food, choose to go down the produce aisle first. This is where all of the fresh fruit and vegetables are. This area should get you excited! Try to eat every fruit and vegetable there is, at least once over your lifespan. You will be thankful if you do this early in life. Think of the different dishes that you can prepare using fruits and vegetables. The dishes can range from salads to smoothies. It's up to you and your creativity when planning meals.

Bread and Cereal

Bread and cereal should be next on your list. Oatmeal for breakfast with low-fat wheat toast sounds delicious! I normally use natural honey to sweeten the oatmeal. The toast that is eaten would be dry. That means no sugar, butter, or anything else. The goal is to find out what you like to eat for breakfast that is healthy for you. You will have to read the labels on cereal boxes to check for the amount of sugar and calories that are in a serving. Eating oatmeal or another natural grain is a smarter choice. Let's just make sure that it's healthy and helps you reach your goals. Again, when you shop for cereal, make sure that the cereal is not loaded with sugar. You have to be a real detective when reading the labels on the packaging box. You will also have to check the amount of calories in the bread.

Dairy and Eggs

When shopping for dairy and eggs, remember to follow the advice and plans that you made with your nutritionist, dietician, or other professional. If you are allergic to certain dairy items, take this into consideration as well. Choose plant-based milk products as an alternative and healthier option to normal milk choices. You will have to make sure that the alternatives are unsweetened. Eggs are a good source of protein and can be used to make a variety of other meals. If you are able to include eggs in your plan, there are good benefits. Eating only the egg whites is a good option.

Nuts and Grains

Nuts and grains are natural and good for you. From rice, beans, barley, and quinoa to pistachios, cashews, peanuts, and walnuts, the variety of food in this area should satisfy your hunger cravings. These foods can be high in fat and calories. So, do not overdo it. These types of food are very good for your heart. They are also a good snack before a game or any occasion.

Frozen Foods and Vegetables

Shopping for frozen food is very difficult. Everything looks so good, but most of it is bad for your health. You have to pay attention to the amount of sodium and calories in the food that you are about to purchase. Frozen vegetables are a good option. The amount of frozen food that you buy when shopping should be carefully considered. You don't want to eat frozen food all of the time. You should strive to eat fresh food as much as possible.

Beverages

High calorie, high sugar, and high caffeine beverages damage health goals. Choose lighter options. Whether it's juice, soda pop, energy drinks, tea, or coffee, decide whether the beverages that you are choosing matches your basketball, health, and fitness goals.

Dry Food and Canned Goods

High sodium and high calories must be checked when shopping for dry foods and canned goods. Read the food labels. Count the number of servings in the can or package as well.

Lean Meats and Seafood

When choosing meats, make sure that the meat fits into your long-term health goals. The meat should be low in fat. Check the label on the package. This includes fish and shellfish. Your dietitian, nutritionist, or other professional should be consulted if you are undecided on what meat to eat or not eat.

Chapter 7

Chapter 7
Dining at Restaurants

Appetizers and Drinks

Imagine the following scenario. You are on a date with your significant other. It's your anniversary. Your intentions are to be conscious of what you are going to eat and drink over the course of the evening, but you want to have fun and enjoy yourself as well. This is a situation that could lead to a person resorting back to bad eating habits because of the instant gratification that's received from not caring about what you eat or drink. To overcome negative self-talk and the impulsive eating of food, a strategic plan should be developed and followed. The plan that's created should outline steps to follow when presented with the urge to eat food without caring about what it is that you are eating or how many calories are in it.

Ordering appetizers, drinks, and food from the menu should be done carefully. Some appetizers could have as many calories in the entire dish than what's required for an individual's daily intake. Beverages and alcoholic drinks can be loaded with sugar and sodium as well. Sharing the appetizers that you select at a restaurant is a good choice. It helps you to reduce the amount of calories that you take in. It also may improve the conversation that you have with the guest that you are sharing the food with. Make sure to ask about the ingredients that are used to make the beverage that you order. You may be surprised at what's in it.

Low Sugar, Low Sodium, Low Calorie Options

The menu choices at the restaurant that you dine at should have information about the amount of calories that are in an entree. Low sugar, low sodium, and low-calorie food entrees should be prioritized over those that are high calorie, full of grease and fat. Carefully monitor your calorie intake during this time. The food that you order will taste so good that you may want to eat more. Don't overeat. Take smaller bites out of your food so that it will last. This may be hard to do as you are sitting there, and the smell of grilled food is in the air, causing you to eat and want more food. You also may be preoccupied in a conversation and don't realize that you are eating too much. Please be cautious of how much you eat.

At some restaurants, the amounts of calories that are in a food item are not given. The portion size that you have ordered may be doubled. If you are unsure of the amount of calories in your food or portion size, just simply ask the waiter or waitress that is helping you. Taking these cautious steps will help you reach your training goals. Start by checking the amount of calories in your favorite foods. If the amount of calories that are in your favorite foods at the restaurant does not surprise you, then try looking at other food items that you would normally eat. These small steps will help you become an informed and health-conscious individual.

Choosing Healthy Replacement Options

There may be times when you visit a restaurant and order a dish that has a side item on it that you do not like or want. You have the choice to replace it with anything that you want. When this occurs, choose to replace the side dish with vegetables or fruit. These are healthy options that won't pack on pounds. Food has a way of changing your mood. Especially when you are eating dessert entrees. When it's time to select a dessert to eat, remember to watch for high sugar desserts and do not choose those desserts to eat. The dessert you choose can also be shared with someone. Overall, when dining at a restaurant, being careful not to eat or drink too much is the key to reaching your training goals.

What happens when you are asked question after question by the person or people that you are dining with about your selective behavior when ordering food? You can explain your plan to them or discuss a similar topic about your wanting to diet and make a change in your eating habits. The person or people that you are with will normally reply by agreeing with you and how they are trying to make changes. This may not be the case all of the time. If you end up having dinner with someone that just simply laughs or berates your choices, then make the choice to not dine with that person again. It will help you in the long run. You want to be around people that will support and encourage you.

Chapter 8

Chapter 8
Snack Foods

The industry is booming. Snack foods are popular and everywhere. From sporting events to family gatherings, snack foods are present and reign supreme. So, what are snack foods exactly? Well, snack foods are any food item that is packaged individually or in bulk and is readily available to be consumed by an individual. Examples of snack foods are packaged chips, cookies, candy, yogurt, cheese, breakfast bars, granola bars, crackers, meat, etc. The amount of snack foods that's consumed on a daily basis by an individual can cause their daily calorie intake to skyrocket out of control. The food that is packaged may be high in sodium, sugar, or fat. Not all snack food is bad. There are some snack foods that are packed with nutrients and ingredients that a person needs on a daily basis. However, the serving size of the snack foods varies from package to package, so individuals could sometimes be eating two times the servings of a particular snack food. The quick and easy access to purchase the food item is what makes snack foods popular. Look at the checkout lines at retail stores. They are normally aligned with candy and snack foods near the checkout line. It becomes a replacement meal that can be eaten at any time of the day. Commercials and Ads bombard us daily with the newest snack foods and beverages. The temptation to try food that's appealing to the eye and is sweet takes over a person's emotions. Not being able to control emotions when craving a certain snack food is a problem that should be solved. Most athletes today face the challenge of not eating meals that are healthy enough to provide nutritional value to their long-term growth and health. They decide to eat snack foods the majority of the time. The breakdown of the family basically starts here. When there is no time to eat as a family, snack foods play a major role in filling the gap of what's going to be for dinner. Obesity becomes a problem for athletes because of the constant eating of snack foods over the course of the day. For example, an athlete may eat a breakfast bar and a large bag of chips for breakfast, then eat cookies for lunch, and for dinner, they'd eat candy, a granola bar, and more chips. If you add a soda pop or energy drink to what they ate, then this would be a perfect storm. The way an athlete chooses to manage their consumption of snack foods is important. They are building a foundation for their entire adulthood. So, the plan that is created should map out their season goals as well as goals for their life.

Overpriced Snack Foods

Overpriced snack foods put a dent in your wallet. Let's say for example you buy a large bag of chips and a pack of cookies. You are paying about five dollars for these two items. If a person ate these two items on a daily basis, then they would have spent thirty-five dollars in one week. In a month's time, that's one hundred and forty dollars. In one year, that's one thousand, six hundred and eighty dollars. If a person does this continuously for ten years, then it's $16,800. Now, I know you would probably say that no one would eat chips and cookies for ten years straight on a daily basis. That's correct. However, the amount spent on snack foods by an individual could reach to about five dollars a day.

Chapter 9

Chapter 9
Eating Food to Gain or Lose Weight

Your workout goals require commitment to a carefully planned diet. If your goal is to lose weight, don't attempt fad diets where certain nutrients that your body needs are missing from the daily servings of foods. Develop a clear start and end date for your weight loss goal. In order for you to reach your goals in basketball and life, consideration must be given to how losing the weight that you plan on losing affects your short and long-term health. Said in a different way, find out if losing too much weight in a short amount time affects your long-term health. Get opinions from several doctors or other health professionals to assist you.

When athletes eat food to rapidly gain weight, they are unconsciously sacrificing their long-term health for athletic gratification now. As an individual ages over the years, it becomes harder to consistently take action and participate in daily workouts and follow a nutrition plan. An example of the thought process that an athlete may have when it comes to eating to rapidly gain weight is, "I will gain the weight for the season, then lose it when it's over." The problem with this is there is no consideration on the rapid gain or loss of weight. There is no consideration on what food is eaten. Normally, every and anything is eaten to pack on pounds, and drastic actions are then taken to lose the weight when it's not needed anymore.

There are certain foods that an individual can eat in order to gain weight. Some of the foods are:

Peanut Butter
Beef
Pork
Chicken
Turkey

Pasta

Candy

Overeating traditional foods or any high-calorie food item that is used to overeat

There are certain foods that an individual can eat in order to lose weight. Some of the foods are:

All vegetables

All fruits

Low-fat food items

Low-calorie food items

Low sugar food items

Low sodium food items

Both hands are normally tied when an individual chooses to rapidly gain weight. Other outside influences are urging the individual to gain the weight. The outside influences could be coaches, trainers, friends, or other individuals that don't have the athlete's best interest in mind. Health considerations when choosing to gain or lose weight is as important as choosing a spouse. The decision that you make could add or decrease your lifespan. Again, there will be distractions. The distractions will be the people that are encouraging you to gain or lose weight for competition purposes only. Much effort has to be given to planning and listening to questions and opinions of several knowledgeable health professionals that have your long-term health goals in mind. This should be done before deciding on a new diet plan. Your long-term health goals and plans should be the deciding factor in any decision that has to be made.

Chapter 10

Chapter 10
After Your Playing Career is Finish

Accepting the Next Chapter in Life

Ahh.... You made it! The time has come. You never thought the day would come. Over and over, you have told yourself, "I'm never gonna stop playing." Well, it's true you won't ever stop playing the game that you love, but it's now a new chapter. The new rule for competing at an elite level in basketball entails preparing your body for changes that it's about to experience over the next few years and beyond. You are now older, wiser, and may have aches on some parts of your body. What you eat and how much of what you eat will affect your immediate and long-term health. Eating healthy and smart is important now more than ever. Think of the goals, dreams, and aspirations that you have for the next 5, 10, 15, 20, and 30 years. Write and outline your plan for accomplishing what you think about. Picture your overall health as it relates to what you are doing at each of the next stages of your life.

Laziness

Lazy behaviors and actions will tend to creep into your daily routine. You will say to yourself, "I deserve this after all of those years of working out and sticking to a diet to stay in shape; I'm gonna eat whatever I want, whenever I want." This is the start of a disaster if you choose to act in this manner. To find out if this is true or not, just look around at a friend or an athlete that has been retired for 5-10 years. Have they gained a considerable amount of weight? Do they do things that they once were opposed to doing? I'm not saying that an individual has to constantly be eating healthy food and follow an extremely strict diet. I'm saying that you should have an overall awareness of what you are eating and a plan of action that will keep you on course to meet your long-term goals after your basketball playing career has come to an end. Stay motivated and find other sports and hobbies that will keep you active and wanting to train and prepare. I chose to run in a marathon. You may choose something different.

Lack of a Workout Routine

When there is no daily or weekly workout routine, a retired athlete gets trapped between having too much free time and attending too many events where food is present. When there is free time on hand, the retired athlete may overindulge in drinking alcoholic beverages, eating unhealthy food, and lounging around. When there are events to attend, the retired athlete may overindulge in drinking alcoholic beverages, eating unhealthy food, and sometimes staying out too late. To overcome these problems, view your goals daily and find a workout partner that will keep you motivated. Meet with your medical doctor to make sure that your overall diet plan matches your long-term health goals. Also, work with a dietitian or other professional to help you reach success.

When attending social events when you are a retired athlete, there will be a ton of food at some of the events. Below are descriptions of some of the actions that should be monitored:

1. Eating on Impulse- Imagine you just got to an event and the smell of a certain food takes you on a journey to eating whatever is in sight. You begin to eat food that you said that you were not going to eat.

2. Overeating- One plate is not enough. You may have eaten too fast, and everyone else at your table is still eating. Plus, the food may have been the best that you've had in a while.

3. Eating at Events- you are at a game as a spectator. The smell of food and beverages takes over your sense. Your craving for the food is now at an all-time high.

4. Desserts & Sweets- it starts out with a small bite or piece. Then bite by bite, you become a victim of the dessert that you eat. You eat it

at the event, and then you have to have it again, so you purchase the dessert to take home.

You have accomplished a lot over the course of your basketball career. The next chapter along your journey now requires you to train differently. Gain an understanding of the changes that are happening to your body and accept it. Develop your plan of action and stick to it. You will win!

Chapter 11

Chapter 11
Eating for Longevity

<u>Know and Learn from your Family History</u>

A path has been paved for you. There are messages all along the path. Family members have had addictions, diseases, allergies, and other ailments that affect an individual's health. For example, if you know that diabetes is a major health problem in your family history, then this should make you more health-conscious in this area. If a person is able to know and learn their family's health history, it will cause the person to choose healthier food options as well as become a role model for future generations. This means avoiding certain types of foods, alcoholic beverages, drugs, and ways of life. This is done because of the awareness of the long-term damage to the body and mind that the continued use would cause.

One way to find alternative food options when deciding what to eat for longevity, an individual should consider studying people who have lived a long, healthy, and active lifestyle. There is a certain plan of action that has already been created and followed by a person that has lived a long, healthy, and active lifestyle. Try to obtain a clear understanding of why certain foods are chosen to be eaten, and others are avoided. Pay attention to every detail.

<u>Form a Team</u>

Form a team to include your doctor, dietitian, and other health professionals. The health professionals should have your best interest in mind. You have to be clear when talking to them about your long-term goals regarding your health and family history. After consulting with your physician and getting advice, create and follow an exercise plan that will help you in reaching your short and long-term dieting and health goals. An athletic trainer could be used to help you develop an exercise plan. The exercise plan that is designed should complement the diet that is followed and should be done at least three to four times per week.

When eating for longevity, eliminate late night eating completely from your diet. The long-term benefits of getting gainful rest and eating small portions outweigh staying up late and overeating. By not eating late, you don't have to worry about feeling sick because you've eaten too much. It may seem like the longer an individual stays awake at night, the more food cravings they tend to have. Overcome late night cravings by eating healthy food options and eating them often (breakfast, lunch, dinner) throughout the day. Make sure you drink the correct amount of servings of water each day. It's detrimental to your long-term success.

There was a time during my youth when we had to eat everything on our plates before we could drink water. It took me several years well into my adulthood to learn that drinking water is important and should be done whenever you choose. Basically, I was going off of what was taught by my ancestors. I had to shake the root and change it.

What types of foods should you eat for breakfast, lunch, and dinner? Low sugar, low sodium, low calorie, and low-fat food items are king. The foods in these categories will fuel your body as well as fight off certain diseases that are associated with high calorie, high fat, high sodium, high sugar, and junk foods. Grains, fruits, beans, and vegetables are examples of foods to eat for longevity. Eating small portion sizes and making sure that you do not overeat is important. Eating the right foods for longevity and making good decisions each day will help you benefit long term. Stay committed to reaching your goals!

Chapter 12

Chapter 12
Basketball Diet Strategy

Overview

Basketball Diet a 30-day diet that focuses on eating the right foods for Longevity and In & Out of Season Competition. The key principles of the diet are eating foods that are low in sugar, sodium, fat, and calories. There are three (3) guides that an individual can follow. They are: Personal Plan, During Competition Plan, and Longevity Plan.

Each plan (except for the During Competition Plan) begins with fasting. That is, eating absolutely nothing except water and a multivitamin for 24 to 48 hours. It follows with a period of when there is absolutely no sugar consumed. Reading food labels is very important during this stage. Exercising and drinking water are other components within the Basketball Diet. No late-night eating after 10 pm is allowed when following the Basketball Diet.

Basketball Diet Principles

Check the food labels on every food item you consume.

What to Eat:

- Low Sugar Foods (0-5 grams)
- Low Sodium Foods
- Low-Fat Foods
- Low-Calorie Foods
- Fruits & Vegetables
- Small Portion Sizes
- Beans & Grains

- Water

- Multivitamin

- Lean Meats (optional)

- Lean Fish (optional)

What to Avoid:

- Cigarettes (All types including e-cigarettes)

- Illegal Drugs (Including Marijuana)

- High-Calorie Foods

- High Sodium Foods

- High Fat Foods

- Drinking too much alcohol (more than three glasses daily)

Key Actions:

- No Late-Night Eating or Drinking (after 10 pm; only water)

- Create a Short Term Eating Goal (2 weeks- 1 month)

- Create a Long-Term Eating Goal (1 month or longer)

- Exercise or Fitness Workout 3-4 days per week

- Build a Health Professional Team

- Drink Water Daily

- Take a Multivitamin Daily

Personal Plan Overview

1st Day (24 hours) Fast: No food at all. Only water and a multivitamin.

Days 2-15: No Sugar

Days 16-30: Follow Basketball Diet Principles

Note:

*These are the author's views. Check with a health professional before starting the Basketball Diet.

*If training for competition, increase fruit, vegetables, grains, beans, and water intake. Consult your physician or other health professional for assistance.

Personal Plan

*The weekly Basketball Diet focus for the main dish that is prepared for dinner is listed daily.

*Repeat plan after 30 days

	Sun	Mon	Tues	Wed	Thur	Fri	Sat
Week 1	FAST	Follow All Basketball Diet Principles NO SUGAR Main Dinner Focus: Low Sodium	Follow All Basketball Diet Principles NO SUGAR Main Dinner Focus: Low Sodium	Follow All Basketball Diet Principles NO SUGAR Main Dinner Focus: Low Sodium	Follow All Basketball Diet Principles NO SUGAR Main Dinner Focus: Low Sodium	Follow All Basketball Diet Principles NO SUGAR Main Dinner Focus: Low Sodium	Follow All Basketball Diet Principles NO SUGAR Main Dinner Focus: Low Sodium
Week 2	Follow All Basketball Diet Principles NO SUGAR Main Dinner Focus: Low Fat	Follow All Basketball Diet Principles NO SUGAR Main Dinner Focus: Low Fat	Follow All Basketball Diet Principles NO SUGAR Main Dinner Focus: Low Fat	Follow All Basketball Diet Principles NO SUGAR Main Dinner Focus: Low Fat	Follow All Basketball Diet Principles NO SUGAR Main Dinner Focus: Low Fat	Follow All Basketball Diet Principles NO SUGAR Main Dinner Focus: Low Fat	Follow All Basketball Diet Principles NO SUGAR Main Dinner Focus: Low Fat
Week 3	Follow All Basketball Diet Principles	Follow All Basketball Diet Principles	Follow All Basketball Diet Principles	Follow All Basketball Diet Principles	Follow All Basketball Diet Principles	Follow All Basketball Diet Principles	Follow All Basketball Diet Principles

	NO SUGAR Main Dinner Focus: Low Calorie	Main Dinner Focus: Low Calorie	Main Dinner Focus: Low Calorie	Main Dinner Focus: Low Calorie	Main Dinner Focus: Low Calorie	Main Dinner Focus: Low Calorie	Main Dinner Focus: Low Calorie
Week 4	Follow All Basketball Diet Principles Main Dinner Focus: Low, Sugar, Sodium, Fat, & Calorie	Follow All Basketball Diet Principles Main Dinner Focus: Low, Sugar, Sodium, Fat, & Calorie	Follow All Basketball Diet Principles Main Dinner Focus: Low, Sugar, Sodium, Fat, & Calorie	Follow All Basketball Diet Principles Main Dinner Focus: Low, Sugar, Sodium, Fat, & Calorie	Follow All Basketball Diet Principles Main Dinner Focus: Low, Sugar, Sodium, Fat, & Calorie	Follow All Basketball Diet Principles Main Dinner Focus: Low, Sugar, Sodium, Fat, & Calorie	Follow All Basketball Diet Principles Main Dinner Focus: Low, Sugar, Sodium, Fat, & Calorie
Week 5	Follow All Basketball Diet Principles Main Dinner Focus: Low Sodium	Follow All Basketball Diet Principles Main Dinner Focus: Low Sodium					

During Competition Plan Overview

Days 1-15: No Sugar

Days 16-30: Follow Basketball Diet Principles

Note:

*These are the author's views. Check with a health professional before starting the Basketball Diet.

*If training for competition, increase fruit, vegetables, grains, beans, and water intake. Consult your physician or other health professionals for assistance.

*Do not fast at all when following the During Competition Plan

During Competition Plan

*The weekly Basketball Diet focus for the main dish that is prepared for dinner is listed daily.

*Repeat plan after 30 days

	Sun	Mon	Tues	Wed	Thur	Fri	Sat
Week 1	Follow All Basketball Diet Principles NO SUGAR Main Dinner Focus: Low Sodium	Follow All Basketball Diet Principles NO SUGAR Main Dinner Focus: Low Sodium	Follow All Basketball Diet Principles NO SUGAR Main Dinner Focus: Low Sodium	Follow All Basketball Diet Principles NO SUGAR Main Dinner Focus: Low Sodium	Follow All Basketball Diet Principles NO SUGAR Main Dinner Focus: Low Sodium	Follow All Basketball Diet Principles NO SUGAR Main Dinner Focus: Low Sodium	Follow All Basketball Diet Principles NO SUGAR Main Dinner Focus: Low Sodium
Week 2	Follow All Basketball Diet Principles NO SUGAR Main Dinner Focus: Low Fat	Follow All Basketball Diet Principles NO SUGAR Main Dinner Focus: Low Fat	Follow All Basketball Diet Principles NO SUGAR Main Dinner Focus: Low Fat	Follow All Basketball Diet Principles NO SUGAR Main Dinner Focus: Low Fat	Follow All Basketball Diet Principles NO SUGAR Main Dinner Focus: Low Fat	Follow All Basketball Diet Principles NO SUGAR Main Dinner Focus: Low Fat	Follow All Basketball Diet Principles NO SUGAR Main Dinner Focus: Low Fat
Week 3	Follow All Basketball Diet Principles	Follow All Basketball Diet Principles	Follow All Basketball Diet Principles	Follow All Basketball Diet Principles	Follow All Basketball Diet Principles	Follow All Basketball Diet Principles	Follow All Basketball Diet Principles

	Main Dinner Focus: Low Calorie	Main Dinner Focus: Low Calorie	Main Dinner Focus: Low Calorie	Main Dinner Focus: Low Calorie	Main Dinner Focus: Low Calorie	Main Dinner Focus: Low Calorie	Main Dinner Focus: Low Calorie
Week 4	Follow All Basketball Diet Principles	Follow All Basketball Diet Principles	Follow All Basketball Diet Principles	Follow All Basketball Diet Principles	Follow All Basketball Diet Principles	Follow All Basketball Diet Principles	Follow All Basketball Diet Principles
	Main Dinner Focus: Low Sugar, Sodium, Fat, & Calorie	Main Dinner Focus: Low Sugar, Sodium, Fat, & Calorie	Main Dinner Focus: Low Sugar, Sodium, Fat, & Calorie	Main Dinner Focus: Low Sugar, Sodium, Fat, & Calorie	Main Dinner Focus: Low Sugar, Sodium, Fat, & Calorie	Main Dinner Focus: Low Sugar, Sodium, Fat, & Calorie	Main Dinner Focus: Low Sugar, Sodium, Fat, & Calorie
Week 5	Follow All Basketball Diet Principles	Follow All Basketball Diet Principles					
	Main Dinner Focus: Low Sodium	Main Dinner Focus: Low Sodium					

Longevity Plan Overview

Days 1-2 (48 hours) Fast: No food at all. Only water and a multivitamin.

Days 3-30: No Sugar

Days 31-60: Follow Basketball Diet Principles

Note:

*These are the author's views. Check with a health professional before starting the Basketball Diet.

*If training for competition, increase fruit, vegetables, grains, beans, and water intake. Consult your physician or other health professionals for assistance

Longevity Plan

*The weekly Basketball Diet focus for the main dish that is prepared for dinner is listed daily.

*Repeat plan after 60 days

Month 1

	Sun	Mon	Tues	Wed	Thur	Fri	Sat
Week 1	FAST	FAST	Follow All Basketball Diet Principles NO SUGAR Main Dinner Focus: Low Sodium	Follow All Basketball Diet Principles NO SUGAR Main Dinner Focus: Low Sodium	Follow All Basketball Diet Principles NO SUGAR Main Dinner Focus: Low Sodium	Follow All Basketball Diet Principles NO SUGAR Main Dinner Focus: Low Sodium	Follow All Basketball Diet Principles NO SUGAR Main Dinner Focus: Low Sodium
Week 2	Follow All Basketball Diet Principles NO SUGAR Main Dinner Focus: Low Fat	Follow All Basketball Diet Principles NO SUGAR Main Dinner Focus: Low Fat	Follow All Basketball Diet Principles NO SUGAR Main Dinner Focus: Low Fat	Follow All Basketball Diet Principles NO SUGAR Main Dinner Focus: Low Fat	Follow All Basketball Diet Principles NO SUGAR Main Dinner Focus: Low Fat	Follow All Basketball Diet Principles NO SUGAR Main Dinner Focus: Low Fat	Follow All Basketball Diet Principles NO SUGAR Main Dinner Focus: Low Fat
Week 3	Follow All Basketball Diet Principles	Follow All Basketball Diet Principles	Follow All Basketball Diet Principles	Follow All Basketball Diet Principles	Follow All Basketball Diet Principles	Follow All Basketball Diet Principles	Follow All Basketball Diet Principles

	NO SUGAR Main Dinner Focus: Low Calorie	NO SUGAR Main Dinner Focus: Low Calorie	NO SUGAR Main Dinner Focus: Low Calorie	NO SUGAR Main Dinner Focus: Low Calorie	NO SUGAR Main Dinner Focus: Low Calorie	NO SUGAR Main Dinner Focus: Low Calorie	NO SUGAR Main Dinner Focus: Low Calorie
Week 4	Follow All Basketball Diet Principles NO SUGAR Main Dinner Focus: Low Sugar, Sodium, Fat, & Calorie	Follow All Basketball Diet Principles NO SUGAR Main Dinner Focus: Low Sugar, Sodium, Fat, & Calorie	Follow All Basketball Diet Principles NO SUGAR Main Dinner Focus: Low Sugar, Sodium, Fat, & Calorie	Follow All Basketball Diet Principles NO SUGAR Main Dinner Focus: Low Sugar, Sodium, Fat, & Calorie	Follow All Basketball Diet Principles NO SUGAR Main Dinner Focus: Low Sugar, Sodium, Fat, & Calorie	Follow All Basketball Diet Principles NO SUGAR Main Dinner Focus: Low Sugar, Sodium, Fat, & Calorie	Follow All Basketball Diet Principles NO SUGAR Main Dinner Focus: Low Sugar, Sodium, Fat, & Calorie
Week 5	Follow All Basketball Diet Principles NO SUGAR Main Dinner Focus: Low Sodium	Follow All Basketball Diet Principles NO SUGAR Main Dinner Focus: Low Sodium					

64

Longevity Plan

Month 2

	Sun	Mon	Tues	Wed	Thur	Fri	Sat
Week 5	Follow All Basketball Diet Principles NO SUGAR Main Dinner Focus: Low Sodium	Follow All Basketball Diet Principles NO SUGAR Main Dinner Focus: Low Sodium	Follow All Basketball Diet Principles Main Dinner Focus: Low Sodium	Follow All Basketball Diet Principles Main Dinner Focus: Low Sodium	Follow All Basketball Diet Principles Main Dinner Focus: Low Sodium	Follow All Basketball Diet Principles Main Dinner Focus: Low Sodium	Follow All Basketball Diet Principles Main Dinner Focus: Low Sodium
Week 6	Follow All Basketball Diet Principles Main Dinner Focus: Low Fat	Follow All Basketball Diet Principles Main Dinner Focus: Low Fat	Follow All Basketball Diet Principles Main Dinner Focus: Low Fat	Follow All Basketball Diet Principles Main Dinner Focus: Low Fat	Follow All Basketball Diet Principles Main Dinner Focus: Low Fat	Follow All Basketball Diet Principles Main Dinner Focus: Low Fat	Follow All Basketball Diet Principles Main Dinner Focus: Low Fat
Week 7	Follow All Basketball Diet Principles Main Dinner Focus: Low Calorie	Follow All Basketball Diet Principles Main Dinner Focus: Low Calorie	Follow All Basketball Diet Principles Main Dinner Focus: Low Calorie	Follow All Basketball Diet Principles Main Dinner Focus: Low Calorie	Follow All Basketball Diet Principles Main Dinner Focus: Low Calorie	Follow All Basketball Diet Principles Main Dinner Focus: Low Calorie	Follow All Basketball Diet Principles Main Dinner Focus: Low Calorie
Week 8	Follow All Basketball Diet Principles	Follow All Basketball Diet Principles	Follow All Basketball Diet Principles	Follow All Basketball Diet Principles	Follow All Basketball Diet Principles	Follow All Basketball Diet Principles	Follow All Basketball Diet Principles

	Main Dinner Focus: Low Sugar, Sodium, Fat, & Calorie	Main Dinner Focus: Low Sugar, Sodium, Fat, & Calorie	Main Dinner Focus: Low Sugar, Sodium, Fat, & Calorie	Main Dinner Focus: Low Sugar, Sodium, Fat, & Calorie	Main Dinner Focus: Low Sugar, Sodium, Fat, & Calorie	Main Dinner Focus: Low Sugar, Sodium, Fat, & Calorie	Main Dinner Focus: Low Sugar, Sodium, Fat, & Calorie
Week 9	Follow All Basketball Diet Principles Main Dinner Focus: Low Sodium	Follow All Basketball Diet Principles Main Dinner Focus: Low Sodium					

Notes

Notes

Notes

Notes

70

Notes

Notes

Notes

Notes

Notes

Notes

Notes

Notes

www.ingramcontent.com/pod-product-compliance
Lightning Source LLC
Chambersburg PA
CBHW062121040426
42336CB00041B/2150